HIGHER GROUND

HIGHER GROUND

An Essential Guide for Emerging Healthcare Leaders

SCOTT NELSON

Higher Ground

Published in the United States of America by Summit Leadership Strategies LLC.
Cover design by Erika Duran.

Identifiers:

979-8-9953138-0-9 (Paperback)
979-8-9953138-1-6 (E-Book)

CONTENTS

Dedication

This leadership book, *Higher Ground,* is dedicated to those with the courage to answer the call to leadership: The difference makers. The influencers. The ones on a continuous path of learning, growth, and connection to better themselves, their departments, their organizations, their communities, and beyond...

May your journey be purposeful and impactful, full of importance and meaning.

Here's to you!

Happy journeying...

Cheers!
Scott Nelson

FOREWORD

This book is for all healthcare leaders. And though it focuses heavily on emerging leaders, my hope is that the entirety will resonate with new as well as seasoned professionals. My experiences manifest in the healthcare setting, though through time and experience, I have come to understand that leadership transcends titles, industries, and genres. So often is the case in our fast-paced industries that new leaders are thrust into vacant positions with little to no training. Without the proper training, guidance, mentorship, and support, many will think they have failed and leave their positions prematurely. Today's healthcare industry is more complex, fast-paced, and dynamic than ever before. From pandemics to staffing shortages, new technologies and information systems, healthcare leaders are challenged with managing resources, culture, finances, and the unexpected to provide higher-quality care at lower costs. It is essential that we recruit, train, mentor, and provide the necessary support to our emerging leaders for not only their success but that of our teams, departments, organizations, and communities.

Physician burnout took center stage just a few years ago, and now, with new demands and challenges in the industry, burnout among all caregivers has become a hot topic. In the last several years, it has been reported that approximately twenty percent of healthcare workers have left the industry, creating a massive shortage coupled with Baby Boomer retirements. Recruitment and retention are of the utmost concern for organizations to establish a talented group of individuals who care for our patients, our communities, and the overall health of our society.

This book guides leaders—both new to healthcare and experienced in the industry—to help focus on the essentials for success. By connecting purpose and meaning with an underlying foundation of the organization's values, leaders will find great success navigating the complexities of our modern-day healthcare systems. Having served in the healthcare industry for over twenty years, I have discovered healthcare is a gift that allows us to rise above personal differences regardless of background, political views, sexual orientation, or religious views, to care for all without bias. When we connect to our mission, vision, and values and are present with the needs of the person in front of us, we reach an elevated state of flow and experience the unexpected return of positive energy for the care we provide; I call this *the gift*.

My experience has proven to me that those leaders and departments that purposefully commit to the mission, vision, and values daily will consistently rise to that level of excellence.

Higher Ground is committed to personalizing the experience and promoting strategies that consistently build positive and safe cultures to remain resilient in the ever-complex healthcare industry. Over time, these lessons help guide healthcare leaders to success and can act as a compass for all sectors by drawing on the strengths of their foundations while focusing and committing daily to the mission, vision, and values.

FOR THE BRIDGE BUILDERS

Take a moment and think about the word *mentor*. Who was your greatest mentor? How did they influence your life? What actions have you taken based on the lessons they taught you? What obstacles or barriers did they help remove? What opportunities did they provide? Throughout life, if we're lucky, we'll have one or two mentors that play a significant role in the people and leaders we become. I call these people the bridge builders, and I challenge you on your journey of leadership, if you have not already, to become a bridge builder yourself.

Bridges play a significant role in our world in helping us get to where we need to be. The first bridges were fallen trees and stepping stones, pathways for our ancestors to explore the unknown, a new beginning, a better future, a new life. Symbolically, bridges represent communication, union, human ingenuity, hope, a way to overcome obstacles. Sometimes those obstacles are physical: a deep canyon, a river, a mountain pass. In my state of Oregon, there are over eight thousand bridges creating pathways to our destinations and back, a manifestation of mind over matter. There are invisible bridges too. These are much harder to see. If you look and listen closely, you will recognize the bridge builders. The ones that helped you find your path and removed those barriers to realize a future unimagined.

The question remains: What does it take to be a great leader? What does it take to create a better tomorrow? Maybe a community built on purpose, respect, inclusion, hope, faith, ingenuity, or communion. Maybe understanding our past, the things we did right, and the missteps along the way. Maybe some amends and forgiveness without forgetting or turning away from others' pain. Maybe purposeful effort, time, and commitment. And maybe a choice to be bridge builders, to be leaders, historians, visionaries, mentors, and removers of obstacles. And maybe that choice to lead will create new possibilities. And maybe the time we commit will give us, our caregivers, our patients, and our communities even more than we ever imagined. What bridges are you—are *we*—working on right now? What bridges have we only thought about? Whose help do we need along the way in creating our visions? Considering time, the one thing we can never get back, when will we start? Can we afford to wait? Tomorrow? Next week? Next month? Next year? Or maybe, just maybe, we could simply agree to start today.

I wish you a fantastic journey on your path of leadership and hope that the lessons through *Higher Ground* will help guide your way and add tools to your kit to become an influential culture builder.

MISSION, VISION, AND VALUES

Connecting to a Higher Purpose

Every organization has a carefully designed mission, vision, and values statement to help guide its leaders and employees toward success and the organization's ultimate goals. The mission statement helps identify and define why the company exists and its higher purpose, while the vision statement serves as an aspirational statement of what the organization wants to achieve. The values help guide actions and behavior to ensure the mission and vision are attainable. All three statements are at the heart of the organization and supported by a foundation of values.

So, what distinguishes a good company from a great company? Consistency is part of the equation to greatness: consistency in practice and patient care, consistency in communication, and consistency in the treatment of employees. We could add many other initiatives to the list, but first we must recognize that an organization that only has mission, vision, and values statements in words and not action will fall short of its aspirations and will also fall short in inspiring its employees to reach their full potential.

Question: Do we live our values, or are they just words? Are they just words that an executive team and board members developed during a day of seminar, or are they fully integrated into the internal workings and magic of the organization? Do the employees know the mission, vision, and values of the organization? Do leaders and employees understand how their roles tie into the company's higher purpose and help contribute to the mission? Do leaders and employees know the organization's values and how these values provide the foundation for all the work combined to accomplish the mission and vision of the company? Everyone in the organization—every role—plays a significant part in achieving these higher goals and providing service to the community. It is creating this level of connectivity that elevates organizations to the highest levels of excellence.

This kind of manifestation results from purposeful and concentrated efforts to see the mission, vision, and values actualized to the highest degree. For years, I have challenged my employees to recommit to the mission, vision, and values every day when they enter the building. We are human and are prone to mistakes.

Sometimes, our frustrations get the best of us, and we disrespect a colleague. There will be times when we get so caught up in our tasks that we fail to show as much compassion as a situation demands. Sometimes we get overwhelmed with the amount of work before us and fail to hold ourselves and others accountable. Understanding our humanity allows us to have the humility to recognize the importance of recommitting each day to the organization's mission, vision, and values.

In a sense, it is exhilarating to understand that each day is a new day with endless possibilities for success, positive interactions, and new understandings of how to do things better. If we stay focused, purposeful, and committed to the mission, vision, and values of our organizations, we will find success.

My challenge to myself and all of you as leaders is this: Every day, before you walk into the building, center yourself on the organization's values, the very essence that paves the way for the mission and vision to be accomplished. Hold yourself and others accountable to this, and you will find your organization headed toward the higher ground of excellence where greatness can occur for the organization and for every individual within.

Truly what we all desire is to belong to something larger than ourselves; this holds great importance and meaning and can help another human being. After all, the organization is only as successful as the sum of its parts.

Servant Leadership

In today's healthcare industry, with all the additional stresses, we need to be able to engage our staff in the critical work they are doing. Helping them connect to purpose and meaning helps us stay fresh, rejuvenated, and away from the dangers of burnout. An engaged staff is committed to continuous process improvement. Continuous process improvement leads to better quality and safety. Better quality and safety lead to better outcomes. Better outcomes lead to more successes and financial stability, all based on a foundation of supporting our staff by providing the training, resources, equipment, and process improvement guidance they need to be successful. Our job as leaders is to learn and understand what our staff needs to do their jobs successfully.

Authentic Leadership

Being yourself and allowing others to be themselves in a safe and transparent environment.

Being true to ourselves allows us to be authentic and genuine and meet others where they are. I have always said we must speak our truths, provide data as supporting evidence, and stay positively persistent in the things we believe in order to see them come to fruition. Caregivers respond to authenticity and want leaders who will be honest with them, listen to their frustrations, and help remove barriers to success. Being true to yourself allows you to be true to your team and serve them with honest conversations, positive collaboration, and a culture that promotes the notion that every voice is valuable. Being yourself allows space for others to authentically express themselves.

Huddle Up

Huddles accomplish many positive things for a team. The two most important are information sharing and reminders.

Information Sharing: Huddles are great for covering safety issues, new methods, equipment and supply needs, staffing, information and announcements, and are an opportunity for recognition and good catches. Recognition helps create momentum for teams to recognize the good things happening. This takes some training, as we are preprogrammed as human beings to acknowledge the things that aren't going well to survive. This instinct comes in handy as healthcare workers, as we are great problem solvers, recognize safety problems and concerns immediately, and are quick to implement a fix. But too much focus on the negative can lead us to a place where we miss the good stuff, the stuff that inspires us to keep coming back, the stuff that rejuvenates us and keeps us from burning out. Celebrate the good stuff every day, and you will soon help develop a team that recognizes all the good things happening, which helps build a positive and safe culture.

Reminders: The second thing the daily huddle does is brings us face to face to remind us each day that we are doing this together, that we need to rely on each other, and that we are stronger and more resilient together. A unified team can overcome significant obstacles, will be more resilient, and can accomplish unimaginable things. A group divided will quickly erode the morale and avoid communication and collaboration, resulting in errors and harm to the patient, staff turnover, and ultimate failure in delivering high-quality care.

We have established that consistency is critical in going from a good organization to an excellent one, and it is no different from our work to create a positive and safe culture. Consistent daily huddles structured around safety, methods, equipment, staffing, information, and opportunities to recognize others will align our actions with excellence.

CUSTOMER EXTRAORDINAIRE JOHN

Making a Difference

Making a difference in another's life gives great purpose and meaning to the work we do and the care we provide. So often, the small things make the most significant difference. A warm blanket, a friendly smile, or a kind word can ease a patient's fears and anxieties about the exam or procedure they are about to undergo. One of the simplest things we can do each day to make the world a better place is to acknowledge the presence and worth of another human being simply by being in the moment with them.

My first example is ironically not from the healthcare industry. I'd worked in healthcare for over ten years and as a leader for over five years. Happily married and a father of three, I was juggling the demands of leadership and family life and—like so many of us—was struggling to find a balance.

My forty-five-minute commute allowed me time to unwind from the working day, though some days were harder to let go than others. Being a dedicated caffeine addict, I began to stop by a local fast-food restaurant in the next town on my journey home, and that's where my story with Customer Extraordinaire John begins.

When I first met John, his Southern drawl and hospitality stood slightly out of place in the Pacific Northwest. He was always in the moment, full of positive energy, and addressed me by saying, "Hey, Boss. How's the day going?" Just that simple jest jolted me from my worries to engage in friendly conversation. Each day, when I'd stop through the drive-thru to order my coffee, John would greet me in the same manner.

It endeared him to me that he always addressed me as "Boss," for I was a boss and always striving to be better. Intellectually, I suspected that John addressed everyone he encountered in the drive-thru as "Boss," and still I enjoyed the fact he had no idea I was a boss.

When John wasn't working, I'd find myself comparing the other employees to the standards John had set all by himself, perhaps by his very nature, and I found myself disappointed. In fact, to this day, I have never encountered another fast-food employee who surpasses the exceptional customer service that John exemplified. I started sharing the lessons I was learning from John with my staff; we, as a team, were focused on improving customer service, patient engagement, and satisfaction. As a crew, we realized that the little things could sometimes make the most significant difference.

Then the day came. That magical day when John took customer service to the next level. That evening, as I was pulling into the drive-thru, I felt burned out from the day. Deadlines, caregiver relations, and the current budgetary concerns weighed heavily on me. I desperately needed a cup of java to get me the next twenty miles home.

I pulled up to the mic, and to my disappointment, it wasn't John working the station. Mindlessly, I ordered my large coffee with two creams and waited behind the car in front of me to move forward—and that's when I saw John. He was leaning out of the front window, smiling, and holding up his hand with his index finger pointed as someone would if they were proclaiming they were number one, or perhaps hold on a minute. Puzzled by the gesture, I smiled and waved. When I finally pulled up to the drive-thru window, John leaned out and said, "Hey, Boss. How you doing today?"

"Great," I replied. Only a partial truth with everything I had on my mind.

"I just wanted to tell you that this pot," he said, holding out the coffee pot, "is running low and old, so I'm gonna make you a fresh one. If you don't mind pulling forward to that waiting spot," he said, gesturing, "I'll get it right out to you."

I smiled, thanked John, and pulled forward as instructed. My worries of the day seemed to have flown from my mind. This momentary connection with another human, seemingly with my best interest in mind—after all, he was making me a fresh pot—had lifted my troubles. Now, intuitively, I knew that John wasn't just making the next pot of coffee for me. I also had to admit that he probably addressed everyone as "Boss." Yet despite my intellectual prowess, the interchange created a powerfully positive impact on my day, and I found myself looking forward to my nightly, though brief, discussions with John.

The little things can make the most significant differences in our lives. To this day, I have yet to meet another employee who surpasses John's exceptional customer service.

In healthcare, I wondered what kind of healing was possible if we all consistently did that for our patients.

And if we show that level of compassion for our patients, can we show it for each other?

ASSUMING POSITIVE INTENT

Assuming positive intent is one of the greatest tools I have been given for my kit of influential culture building. I learned about the idea in my first year of leadership. You will make mistakes your entire career, and have areas that you will need to adjust and realign. My own first year as a leader was certainly filled with some serious missteps.

One day, from my office, I saw another leader talking to my crew and giving them instructions on handling a particular situation. I believe it was because I was insecure about many things that I reacted the way I did that first year. Immediately, my ego got in the way and started telling myself a story: *Why was this other leader giving my staff directions without talking to me first? It's my staff, after all.* My emotions soared, and my insecurities got the best of me. I questioned the other leader in front of my staff and stopped the conversation in its tracks. It's probably one of the worst things you can do to another leader or person, and I immediately regretted my approach. After a few minutes, I walked over to her office and apologized. She was receptive, and we discussed the situation and what she was trying to convey to my team. She reassured me that she would never do anything to undermine my leadership.

She should not have had to explain herself to me, but in my first year of leadership, I had many insecurities, and although a vast majority of the time I was aligned with the values of the organization and had compassion and respect for others, this was one time I missed the boat. Fortunately for me, she was a seasoned leader and was able to help me and forgive my transgressions, and we went on to have a strong bond and professional relationship where we could rely on each other to speak our truths with compassion and respect.

In this same first year, my senior leader introduced me to the concept of bringing everything back to the mission, vision, and values and how they related to the patients, the physicians, and each other. Primarily when referring to the patients, she highlighted our initiatives or actions by asking the question, "Is this something the patient would want to pay for? If not, we probably shouldn't be doing it."

During one of our leadership development trainings in my first year of leadership, I was introduced to the concept of positive intent. What is positive intent and how does it free you as an individual? As it was explained, positive intent incorporates the notion that everyone who showed up to work today showed up to do the best job they can. Taking on this perspective frees us from preconceived notions or biases before we truly understand what happened. Assuming positive intent allows one to approach people and ask questions that I usually would not ask if I were assuming negative intent; unfortunately, this happens most of the time. We as human beings see or hear something, and because we need to fill in the gaps of understanding, we immediately jump to a conclusion and believe our judgment to be true when we couldn't be further from the truth. Case in point, I came down hard on the other leader instructing my staff without consulting with me first. My ego got in the way, and since that embarrassing and uncomfortable moment in leadership, I have learned that the better job I do of setting my ego aside and getting out of my own way, the better job I do in supporting, serving, and leading others.

Assuming positive intent allows us, when things go wrong, to go directly to the source, to the person, and ask simple questions to get to the heart of the matter and collaborate for a resolution. It can be as simple as, "Help me understand what happened." By approaching the other person with compassion, respect, and a willingness to understand, we can create powerful situations of resolution and higher understanding. We may indeed be wrong. As I have learned over the years, when I try and guess other people's motivations, I am generally wrong ninety-nine percent of the time.

How often do employees think, *If this other person would just do their job right, my job would be so much easier?* We ask this question to ourselves at best, and at worst, we gossip about the other person, complain to our trusted colleagues about them, and spin up the entire office. Consequently, the other person has no idea there is a problem, and the issue remains unresolved. These situations create a toxic environment and distrust, and result in poor outcomes. So how do we get to a higher level of thinking? A higher level of existing and creating that culture we all want to be part of? By assuming positive intent and going directly to the person to ask the question, have conversations, and positively collaborate for resolution. Staying grounded in our mission, vision, and values and assuming positive intent will permit us to seek resolution, build trusted relationships, and result in creating positive cultures beyond what we previously believed to be possible. If people don't feel comfortable having that conversation alone, if it is not psychologically safe enough, encourage them or yourself to incorporate another leader or Human Resources business partner to help create a safe space for the conversation to take place.

My challenge to you: Next time you walk through the doors of your organization, recommit yourself to the organization's mission, vision, and values, and add assuming positive intent to your tools of influential culture builders and see what happens. I promise that it will transform your life and open new possibilities and opportunities you never dreamed possible. Give it a try. What do you have to lose? How has assuming negative intent, proving others wrong, and gossiping worked out in the past? Assume positive intent and change your life, positively influence the lives of others around you to build the most positive cultures, and produce the best outcomes for your employees and patients.

Now, I would love to tell you that I get this correct one hundred percent of the time, but just like you, I am human, prone to inconsistencies, biases, and mistakes. We, as human beings and leaders, will sometimes get it wrong. During those times, our mission, vision, and values will help get us back on track and realign our commitments to ourselves and others. If you do make mistakes (and you will), try and recognize them quickly and make amends where needed. Even though you made a mistake and possibly disrespected another person, making amends will help build relationships and trust. As leaders committed to authenticity, we must admit when we are wrong.

I must admit that assuming positive intent is a little easier at work than in my personal life. After all, our loved ones—especially if you have children—know how to push our buttons and throw us off our game. I have found that this concept of assuming positive intent is powerful in all aspects and areas of one's life if we can learn to purposefully commit to the idea, go straight to the person, and ask questions for a higher level of understanding. Assuming positive intent frees us up to create these collaborations and can save us a lot of grief and pain if we are willing to try it and purposefully incorporate it into our lives. This concept was gifted to me many years ago and has been a critical strength in finding success as a leader. Make sure this one is in your toolkit.

BUILDING A CULTURE OF TRUST

For any organization to find true success, there needs to be a level of trust established. For those organizations seeking the highest levels of success and excellence, trust must be at the forefront of every interaction. Trust is something that takes time to build and earn and is something so easily eroded. Without trust, individuals, teams, departments, and organizations will fall short of their mission and vision. They'll experience higher turnover, more errors, lower employee engagement, and lower staff morale—among other detrimental consequences to the success of the individuals and the organization.

To understand trust, I challenge us to contemplate how trust is lost. When you think of your organization, where can you identify where trust has been violated or lost? What actions lead to the loss of trust? Can you identify areas where trust was lost and reestablished? How? Can you identify areas where trust was lost, resulting in the loss of employees? If so, what consequences did this pose for your department? For the organization? Personally?

So, how do we lose trust? The following are examples I have witnessed throughout my career:

- Not following the values of the organization
- Inconsistency
- Lack of communication
- Dishonesty
- Words not matching action
- Inability to actively listen to others
- Lack of follow-through
- Inability to admit mistakes
- Not valuing others
- Not including others
- Unwillingness to provide support, mentorship, or leadership

We could continue adding to this list, and if asked, I believe all of us could develop specific examples for each category. As leaders, if we are honest with ourselves, we can probably identify areas where we have contributed to a lack of trust among our employees.

My most extreme example of broken trust involved a department and a Health Insurance Portability and Accountability Act (HIPAA) violation. The occurrence had taken place months before I accepted the position as the director of the department. I would learn details over time about why I had inherited a team divided into three groups. Two groups were at odds with each other and would only speak if there was a work demand; another group was trying to survive and found themselves caught in between.

I almost didn't accept the directorship. For any leadership position, I will only accept if I can answer a few simple questions. One: Why do I want to serve the organization? Two: Why do I want to serve the community? Three: Do I believe I can make a difference?

The interview for the Director of Imaging was an all-day process consisting of an interview with fellow directors, the administrative team, and the radiology department—those whom I would be serving directly. Five years prior, I had worked with most of the department in my specified roles as an X-ray, CT, and MRI technologist. These were my prior colleagues I would be serving after leaving for five years to serve as the Director of Imaging in my first leadership role at a hospital just seventeen miles away from my community.

The interview with the technologists took place in the tech area. I could tell right away that something was wrong. The air was tense as the group struggled to ask me questions. Previously, I had been warned by the Human Resources Director that the group had gone through a difficult time with a HIPAA violation that divided them. It quickly became apparent that the groups did not trust each other and were afraid to ask me a question for fear of being judged silently by their coworkers.

So instead, I started asking them questions. Questions like, "What are you looking for in your ideal candidate?" "What projects and goals do you hope to accomplish this next year?" "What challenges do you think a new leader will experience in the first six months of the position?" I ended up asking questions and offering my answers without being prompted for about forty-five minutes before the Director of HR retrieved me for the final tour of the hospital.

As the director showed me around, I remember thinking that I would not accept the position, knowing that I had to answer two questions to accept. One: Why did I want to serve the community? That question was easy to answer, as I lived in the community and had been commuting for the last five years to my current job seventeen miles away. The other question was much harder to answer: Did I think I could make a difference? After getting a feel for the group and having worked with them prior, I had too many doubts about turning them around and feared I did not have the leadership skills to turn the group into a high-functioning team. After all, this team struggled to even ask me questions at my interview, and they knew me.

That night, when my wife asked me about the position, I told her I didn't think I would accept the offer. Though I wanted to serve the community, I had many doubts about the team. Besides, I'd be leaving the current high-functioning team I loved, a group I had worked hard to purposefully align with the mission, vision, and values after a very tough first year of hard work, struggles, and doubts. Now, after five years of developing into a highly functioning team, I had to ask myself: Why would I leave my team for this new one?

I have to admit, it's easy to get complacent after working hard to put a team together. I was letting my fears and doubts decide for me, and if it hadn't been for an inspirational conversation with the Chief Executive Officer, I would not have accepted the new position. She was in Hawaii at a leadership conference when I had my one-on-one conversation with her about the position. After almost two hours of discussing healthcare philosophy and realizing that our philosophies were aligned and that I had her support in doing whatever I needed to do to realign the team with the mission, vision, and values, I accepted the new position and leaned into the new role without reservations.

The following year would be the most challenging of my leadership career. There were moments of doubt that I had made a mistake and couldn't turn the group around—a group that despised each other and would only talk to each other if a patient was involved, no sharing of life, weekends, celebrations, etc. Restructuring proved necessary, and after three months, I dissolved the two coordinator positions and created leads for each modality to disperse the power dynamics of the department. There was now a lead technologist in CT, ultrasound, nuclear medicine, X-ray, and mammography. We implemented daily huddles focused on safety, quality, managing up, and recognition. I emphasized that the daily huddles served two purposes: 1) To dispense information around safety, equipment, staffing, processes, and recognitions. 2) To remind us each day that we are in this together and need positive collaboration to be successful despite any personal differences or disagreements. By focusing on our primary purpose, taking care of our patients, and realigning with the values of our organization, we slowly, and day by day, started to make a change in our team.

Though we had six values that provided the foundation for our organization (compassion, respect, collaboration, accountability, integrity, and excellence), I started with the first two. I coached my crew that if they could not remember all of the values, to focus on these two first: compassion and respect. I informed them that these values would help them succeed in almost any scenario. No matter what you do, always remember compassion and respect. The next thing I implemented immediately was a patient care initiative to take the negative focus off of each other and focus positive energy on our patients, where our passions aligned.

I have yet to meet a caregiver who is not passionate about patient care and does not have a personalized answer to the question, "What does patient care mean to you?" By focusing on our first two values of compassion and respect, and taking the negative focus off of each other and putting a positive focus on the patient, the crew was beginning to align with the mission, vision, and values of the organization; find common ground; and begin in small ways to function as a team. It would prove to be the most challenging year of my professional leadership career, with doubts along the way. I'd accepted the position to serve my community and make a difference. During moments of doubt, the question ate at my conscience, but I would need to move on. Remaining with the organization would prove to me as a leader that if you stay consistent and authentic to the mission, vision, and values, and hold yourself and others accountable, you can overcome seemingly insurmountable odds and achieve things you never thought possible.

After a year of challenging, purposeful, and committed work, the group developed into a highly functioning team aligned with the mission, vision, and values, and would grow to overcome their differences and learn to enjoy each other's company. I would see employees, who a year earlier would only speak to each other if it involved a common patient, sharing their lives and bonding over life experiences and what they did over their weekends. We had overcome and reached a higher level of understanding and existence, a higher level where we intuitively knew that our differences only held us back from delivering the highest quality of care and reaching a level of excellence. It was our commonalities and shared purpose that would elevate us to this higher level.

Culture of Trust = Culture of Safety

To promote a safe culture, we must first work on trust. Without trust, safety, quality, and morale, our reputation will suffer. So, how do we build trust? The first step to building trust is focusing on our mission, vision, values and our daily commitment to hold ourselves and others accountable. Staying true to the values allows us to work for a common core of expectations and build our professional relationships from this foundation.

Relationship building based on respect and compassion helps us elevate to the higher level of space we need to complete our mission and vision. This action elevates us beyond personalities, differences, and perspectives to a place of genuine commitment to excellence. By being purposeful with these initiatives toward each other, our physicians, and our patients, we can build trust and create cultures that promote open communication, transparency, and honest feedback to highlight quality and safety issues.

A culture where people feel safe to stop the line, bring up safety concerns, and report to a safety alert system from the place of wanting to help improve practices and not from a blame-centric perspective will promote the safest of environments. Historically, healthcare has been a blame industry for medical errors and mistakes, and in some instances, blame is still being bestowed upon employees. However, a blame culture instills fear and inaction and unintentionally results in more errors, safety concerns, and harm to our patients. We must commit to safe cultures where people feel comfortable speaking up and being part of the solution to safer and higher-quality patient care. This type of engagement requires caregiver and physician buy-in and support.

As leaders, there are numerous opportunities to coach, thank, and manage employees willing to speak up, stand up, and report errors or near misses. The near misses that, if left unreported, will most likely end up as an error the next time.

In my early career as an MRI technologist, in my first six months, we had just finished with an inpatient that needed to return to the floor. Our MRI table did not detach at the time, so we kept a nonferromagnetic stretcher in the scan room to transport patients. We moved the patient onto this stretcher and out into the hallway, where we hooked up the oxygen tank outside the MRI room and placed the tank next to the patient. A student technologist and I transported the patient to their floor room, put the oxygen tank under the stretcher, and proceeded back to the MRI suite. On the way back, the student and I got caught up in conversation as we enjoyed the day and shared stories. As we entered the MRI room with the nonferromagnetic stretcher, another senior MRI technologist stopped us just inside the scan room with an abrupt, “Stop!”

She had noticed the oxygen tank under the stretcher, something that could have quickly become dislodged by the MRI magnet, seriously injured or killed one of us, and certainly damaged the MRI magnet itself. Fortunately, the senior technologist stopped us in time.

At first, with adrenaline pumping, we all counted our blessings, got the stretcher outside the scan room, removed the oxygen tank, and then moved the nonferromagnetic stretcher back into the MRI scan room, where we stored it in the back corner. The senior technologists initially said we did not need to report the event because no one was injured. However, after our adrenaline wore off, we realized that was not the proper thing to do, and if left unreported, we were violating several values, including accountability and integrity, and potentially setting up a dangerous future situation. Instead, we did the right thing: We reported the event to our department director as well as the safety reporting system, which allowed us to implement a safer protocol for screening items—including our nonferromagnetic stretcher for any hazardous objects that could be ferromagnetic and cause serious injury to a person or damage to the MRI machine or room if accidentally taken in. Stopping at the door and checking for any safety concerns became our new routine, and we never had another incident again.

In your organization, strive for a culture of safety where blame is not part of the equation. Hold yourself and others accountable for adhering to best practices, and when things do go wrong (near misses occur, errors happen, or harm reaches the patient), work with your risk and safety officer on a root-cause analysis algorithm to understand how to prevent it from happening going forward. Being transparent and open about these issues with the entire team will create a culture of trust, safety, and consistency in producing good outcomes.

As a leader, what I have discovered in over twenty years of reviewing incident reports is that ninety-nine percent of the time, people want to do what is right and safe and produce a good outcome. So often we uncover an incomplete or bad process, undertrained staff, or cultures that have not created enough trust for people to speak up about their safety concerns. It relates to relationship building, being committed to best practices, and avoiding blame culture. Do this, and your organization will rise to the top as exemplary in safety, quality, and great patient outcomes and experiences. Commitment + consistency + transparency + grounded in mission, vision, and values = great outcomes.

COMPASSION AND RESPECT

Remember, I asked my crew that if they couldn't remember all the values right away, to remember these two: compassion and respect. Compassion and respect would provide a solid foundation for finding success in most scenarios. That's right, *most.* Eventually, we will need to incorporate the other four values, but first things first: compassion and respect.

During the first challenging year, I would often ask employees about their perception of their patient care during our one-on-one meetings. Unequivocally, everyone answered the same. Each caregiver believed they provided exceptional care one hundred percent of the time. During these meetings, I would also ask them if they thought their patients could tell they didn't necessarily get along with a coworker. Again, unequivocally, each caregiver believed that patients couldn't tell that they genuinely had a poor relationship, that there were deep resentments and distrust among them, and that they would rather be doing anything else than having to speak to their coworker.

As an outsider looking in, and being a new leader in the department, I knew how wrong and self-deceived they were. Patients watch and listen to everything we do and say to see if they can trust us with their care. They often arrive frightened with a heightened awareness of what might happen. They are looking for reasons to trust us and quickly pick up on anything that doesn't feel right: the tone of voice, a sideways glance, a coworker quick to criticize a fellow employee, or the hospital itself. In healthcare, we are always on. Everything we do and say is on display for our patients to judge and assess if they will trust us with their care. And we can relate to this. After all, haven't we or our family members been patients at one time and in those vulnerable positions where we've been frightened of the unknown? Frightened about what this diagnostic imaging or lab test might find? Frightened that our health may be compromised and our life altered in devastating ways?

The quickest way to build rapport and trust with our patients is to show compassion and respect for one another. So, if you are to ask yourself what compassion and respect look like, what would your answers be? What do we all want from our experiences with others? Especially those healthcare experiences where we are feeling vulnerable and afraid.

Here is an example from the patient's perspective and why our interactions between coworkers matter:

I am here today for some test. Something is not quite right, and I need to find some answers to get back to living.

I don't want to be here.

I'd rather be anywhere else.

I'm concerned with what they might find. My thoughts are racing, and I feel a little sick to my stomach. I have so many unanswered questions. My fight-or-flight responses are kicking into overdrive. I just want to get out of here as quickly as possible, get back to my friends and family, and get back to my life.

From this perspective, you can see how the slightest thing gone wrong between coworkers in front of the patient or within earshot, even standoffish body language, could really unravel the patient's confidence in their care.

Several years ago, I had the privilege to listen to a charismatic CEO speak. Before his talk, I watched as he mingled with the crowd, asking people where they were from, how they were enjoying the conference, and just making small talk to build rapport and make connections—the building blocks of trust.

Soon he took the stage and launched into his talk. The reason he was asked to speak? His hospital thrived over others in a system of multiple hospitals.

Their patient satisfaction and employee engagement increased significantly in just under a year. Turnover was down, process improvement was up, and his hospital financially was striving beyond the others. Everyone, including the system's top administrators, wanted to know his secret.

The truth is the only thing he was doing differently was taking the time (he and his administrative team) to support the frontline caregivers. What tools did they need? What processes were they struggling with? What additional training or support did they need to do their jobs better? What could the administrative team do differently to help support them? And what did the administrative team focus on? Here was the kicker. This CEO's main focus, the entire team's purpose, consisted of only two things: 1) We take care of people's physical needs, and 2) We take care of people's emotional needs.

Said so simply, dissected down to the essence of things, and as a father of three, it hit me: That's our primary purpose. It's always been our main purpose, especially in healthcare where people are often at their most vulnerable. We take care of their physical and emotional needs. We take the time to listen, care, answer questions, and treat through compassion and respect to help heal our patients both physically and emotionally.

As caregivers, if we can do this for our patients, aligning with our mission, vision, and values, then we can do this for each other. And this is the challenge for all of us. The purpose of commitment is key to creating the culture we all want to be part of. By recognizing our shortcomings in these areas of compassion and respect and recommitting each day to the mission, we as individuals, departments, organizations, and systems will strive toward excellence.

When caregivers feel cared for, engagement increases. When engagement increases, more energy flows into process improvement. When process improvement increases, quality and safety improve. When quality and safety improve, patients have better experiences and better outcomes. When patients have better experiences and results, the financial bottom line improves, perpetuating and sustaining the organization and hospital system for today and the future. And this all starts with compassion and respect.

I am a firm believer that this order does not work in reverse. Those organizations that start with the financial bottom line and make decisions from this platform without engaging the other pillars of excellence will descend into a downward spiral of employee disengagement. Disengagement leads to a lack of commitment to the mission, vision, and values. A lack of commitment to the mission, vision, and values leads to relationships and processes unraveling. This, in turn, leads to distrust. Distrust leads to a lack of collaboration. A lack of cooperation leads to safety and quality issues. Safety and quality issues lead to patient dissatisfaction, distrust, and lack of loyalty to the organization. This leads to high turnover in staff, lower volumes, and a deteriorating organization structure and form, significantly reducing the bottom line and the services offered.

So, again, I challenge you. Each day you come into work, when you walk through the doors, when you clock in, recommit to the organization's mission, vision, and values. The values act as our guide to help us along our journey. We are human, after all, and will make mistakes along the way. There will be times when we show a lack of respect or compassion, when our integrity is challenged, or we fail to hold ourselves or others accountable, and when we fail to collaborate positively with others. Our mission, vision, and values will help us get back on track, allow us to make amends readily, and stay true to ourselves, our patients, and each other. If you can't remember all the values at first, or even if your organization has a few different values, always remember compassion and respect. These two values will help you through almost any situation. Almost.

Accountability

I truly believe that accountability is one of the most challenging values to adhere to. There are times as leaders, if we are being honest with ourselves, that we wish we hadn't seen something, heard something, or learned something, as it is those times that we must act or fail to hold ourselves and others accountable. Sometimes, as a human being, you discover something undesirable and want to walk away from it. However, as a leader, we know we must address the issues with compassion and respect for better results.

In my first year of leadership, I heard the phrase often from my mentor, "What you allow, you promote." This quote empowered me to have courage and address the issue even when I just wanted to walk away. Being a leader is not for the faint of heart, and there are times when you must have a crucial conversation with an employee. Sometimes it centers around a mistake, tardiness or absenteeism, behaviors not aligned with the values, or an error that reached the patient.

If done with compassion and respect, almost any situation can be corrected for a better result moving forward. One thing that has helped me as a leader, especially when dealing with Human Resource issues, is to know that I am genuinely rooting for the success of every employee and will do anything in my power to help them succeed. This sometimes involves corrective or disciplinary action. These actions are up to the employee to align with the organization's mission, vision, and values; this is a daily choice.

If the employee chooses not to align, that is their choice with natural consequences to follow that are both known and transparent. In my entire twenty-plus years of being a leader (except for a HIPAA violation that was negligent), I have not encountered a situation with an employee willing to align with the mission, vision, and values that did not result in better outcomes and success for the employee, the department, and the organization.

Remember, coaching is caring. If we are not speaking up and informing our employees when they are outside the expectations of the values, then we are not holding ourselves accountable as leaders and are essentially letting our employees down. Sometimes, the employee isn't even aware of how their actions or behaviors affect others. As I've heard it said by many healthcare leaders, holding others accountable without coaching is cruelty.

As leaders, accountability starts with us. Do we hold ourselves accountable to align with the mission, vision, and values? Do we walk the talk? Do we believe coaching is caring and help bring transparency to our staff? Do we admit our mistakes and make amends where necessary? Do we hold ourselves accountable to our professional organizations, commitments, timelines, projects, patients, employees, physicians, and communities?

You can add your own to the list of accountabilities and what you believe are the highest priorities to fulfill the mission and vision. Here are a couple examples for myself of what it means to walk the talk: 1) I am a firm believer that a clean hospital is a safer hospital, and as an example of accountability, I do not allow myself to walk past a piece of trash on the ground without picking it up. To be an owner means to act as such, and it feels good to put yourself into the situation and be a part of the solution, rather than simply saying it's not my job and walk away. 2) Engage, and you will discover new rewards you had no idea existed. Engage, and you will help lead your teams to new heights of excellence.

Respect

Respect. What does it look like? When respect is missing, you immediately know and feel it in your interactions with others.

It has often been said that respect has to be earned, and in some sense, there is truth in this statement. However, this perspective sets respect up in a competition for action, achievement, and comparisons to others. Respect in the collaborative and supportive sense leads to listening more intently, recognizing when others are not feeling safe, and going out of your way to make others feel comfortable, included, and acknowledged.

Respect comes in kind words, a compassionate deed, and putting others' needs ahead of our own. Some of the most powerful things we do on any given day are to recognize another human being, acknowledge their worth, and celebrate our humanness together.

Retrieving a warm blanket for a patient, taking time to listen to an anxious patient or coworker, and calming ourselves when we feel frustrated to listen to another's point of view are all acts of great compassion and respect.

By demonstrating respect to others, we in turn receive respect back. This mutual respect helps to build connections, relationships, and cultures that value each other's voices. Valuing another's voice promotes a culture of safety where staff are not afraid to speak up and stop the line when there is a potential error and possible harm to the patient. We all want this type of safety culture for ourselves, our loved ones, and our friends when they are receiving care. The little things in life, the kind word, the warm blanket, and the act of listening to another's concerns or fears make the most significant differences in another's life and the road to healing.

When respect is missing, it can have the oppositive effect. We've all seen, experienced, and worked to fight against it when respect is lacking. Case in point: A rude surgeon shows their frustrations toward others in high-stress situations, belittles with rude comments, and dismisses the staff. This is a surgeon that no one wants to work with, and a situation where people will often not speak up to state their concerns about a process, a safety concern, or anything else for fear of public humiliation. If we can recognize these situations, hold each other accountable for our behavior, and make it known that it is unacceptable, we will be well on our way to creating a culture of safety where staff feel supported in stating their truth and working toward better collaboration.

To hold ourselves accountable, we must also uncover what frustrates the surgeon. If we only address the poor behavior without recognizing that there may be a legitimate reason why the surgeon is frustrated and acting out, we will be missing a pivotal opportunity to improve the processes and relationships. We cannot afford to let these issues go in a safety culture. Where respect has been betrayed, we as leaders owe it to our staff and physicians to identify the underlying causes, create transparency, and elevate the conversations and collaborations to a higher level of understanding for the best outcomes. By aligning our behaviors and actions to the mission, vision, and values, we will hold each other to the highest level of respect.

I've come to understand that physicians want essentially four things, the same things we all want for our patients and ourselves: high-quality care for their patients, competent staff, their time respected, and being thanked once in a while. It's the little things that make the most significant difference.

Excellence

I firmly believe that all the other values combined add up to excellence. And to achieve excellence, there is one key ingredient that must be present, and that is consistency in the things we do—consistency in aligning to the mission, vision, and values. Consistency in adhering to the policies and procedures, consistency in being in the moment with our patients, physicians, and each other. Consistency in prioritizing care for others. Consistency in showing compassion and respect for each other. Consistency in holding ourselves and others accountable and committing every day with fresh energy toward our initiatives to achieve our goals and fulfill our mission. Consistency with compassion and respect is the key to developing mediocre teams into teams that exude excellence.

I challenge all of us to review our personal commitments, our team and department commitments, our organizational commitments, and our community commitments to determine where we are lacking in consistency, to identify those opportunities to help remove barriers, and recommit to consistently driving change for the best outcomes.

OWNERSHIP, AUTONOMY, ENGAGEMENT

Ownership

How do we define ownership? What does ownership look like? When you consider your actions within your organization, can you call yourself an owner? Do you hold yourself accountable for what you say you will do and the actions you promised to fulfill?

I once heard a healthcare leader say, "You see it, you touch it, you smell it, you own it." When you're walking down the hallway and see a piece of trash on the floor, do you stop to pick it up, or walk by telling yourself it's someone else's job? When you see a patient lost or confused about where they are going, do you take the time to help them? Or do you walk by telling yourself you are too busy to get involved and it's someone else's job? When you see a defect in the hospital infrastructure—a broken door, a clogged toilet, scuffed wall—do you take ownership and put in a work order, or do you turn a blind eye and carry on with your work?

During my first week as the Director of Imaging, I encountered one of our technologists walking down the hallway, and I asked how he was doing that day. His response? "Only a couple more hours until quitting time." As I walked by, I realized that if I did not find a way to engage this employee, I would lose him. I knew he was a good technologist, and considering the cost of turnover and loss of expertise and knowledge when we lose staff, I started working on a plan to engage him.

I had seen this technologist interact with student technologists, and I knew a couple of things: 1) He liked sharing his knowledge and expertise openly to help the student technologists get better, and 2) He took pride in his work and turned in high-quality images. The next day, I approached the technologist and asked if he had ever thought about being the Student Clinical Advisor. He laughed a little and said he liked working with students but didn't want to deal with all that paperwork. Thinking quickly, I asked him if I was able to get someone else to work on the student schedules and mandatory paperwork the college required, would he be willing to be the designated Student Instructor? He warmed to this idea and agreed to take the students officially under his wing. This was a positive step in reengaging this caregiver.

What happened next? Well, he became the best and most recognized Student Coordinator in the region and was recognized at the college graduations with an award strictly voted on by the students on numerous occasions. Our hospital developed a reputation of being the best hospital for students to learn in; this was not only because we had a great student coordinator, but also because we had an entire team that bought into the concept that we do not hold back for our students, because the students we were teaching today could be working alongside us tomorrow or taking care of our family members or us.

This particular technologist who had recently told me there were only a couple more hours until quitting time never said that phrase again when I asked him how his day was going. He engaged in the work, felt valued and respected, and thrived in his new role. He also became our number one identifier of problems in the hospital that had to do with infrastructure—a broken door, scratched surface, or missing paint—and would take ownership of the defects he saw and turn in a work order to our facilities maintenance team. He started to exemplify what being an owner means and became an example for others to follow. Find ways to engage employees, and you will create authentic ownership.

Autonomy

A simple definition states it as an ability to make independent, informed decisions without coercion. What do employees really want? We've learned that empowering and engaging employees and giving them a voice allows them to take ownership and pride in their work. So, how do we accomplish autonomy?

How often do employees call upon leaders for the answers? Afraid to be criticized or make a mistake, employees often hesitate or refuse to decide without the boss's approval. Historically, top-down leadership served from a hierarchical structure, and leadership based on blame and shame has often frozen employees from engaging in decision making.

In the new era of leadership where employees desire a sense of autonomy, new generations demand a say, and the best outcomes come from positive collaboration across roles with increased communication from top to bottom, bottom to top, and side to side. We as leaders must purposefully encourage employee autonomy, which leads to increased engagement and best outcomes. How do we accomplish this as leaders? By giving up some control, trusting our employees, and getting away from the blame-and-shame cultures of the past.

The simplest way to engage employees is to show them you trust them. When they come to you with a question, it is easy for leaders to provide the answer they believe will solve the problem. However, by answering, we have unintentionally disengaged the employee or at least failed to recognize that the employee may have a creative solution to the problem, which may well be better than our answer. So, the next time an employee asks you a question, instead of providing an answer right away, try asking them how they would suggest solving the problem. Dive into a question period where you give the employee the reins of leadership control, decision making, and follow-through. These actions will encourage further development of the caregiver's autonomy in problem solving and decision making.

Just like our own decisions at times, things don't always work out, and we will have to analyze what went well, what didn't go so well, and what we would do differently next time. This will be the same process with employees who make decisions that do not produce the best outcomes. We must not place blame or shame on these decisions, but rather a safe place to fail fast, discover the next steps, adapt, and move forward in a positive direction. By consistently supporting our staff in this fashion, we will develop a culture of engagement, trust, and creativity that will steadily blossom, grow, and become contagious to the rest of the crew.

By showing our employees that we trust them and allowing them to learn from mistakes, we will be creating a sustainable culture of problem solvers. By modeling this behavior as a leader, you will set the tone and stage for your employees to begin treating each other with trust and respect for autonomy in the workday. The results will produce a highly engaged team that plays off each other's strengths.

There is a revolution in leadership—one where the historical hierarchical structure no longer produces the best results. We must engage in servant leadership grounded in our mission, vision, and values to help support our employees so they can reach their full potential and produce the most favorable results not only for the patient, the employee, the physicians, and leadership, but ultimately for the greater good of the community.

Engagement

During my first role as a leader, one of my colleagues repeatedly said, "It's all about relationships." In my career, over twenty-plus years of leadership, I have found this simple proclamation to be the truth behind great cultures. Engaging in authentic leadership, getting to know your staff and their lives, and creating connections allows us to build trust, support, and positive communication that will produce the best of cultures.

Remember the CEO I referenced previously? The one at the healthcare conference that connected with people before his presentation. He was asked to speak because his hospital—one of many in an extensive system—was striding beyond other hospitals regarding employee engagement, patient satisfaction, and physician satisfaction. Everyone wanted to know what his secret was.

The secret? Making personal connections and building the relationships from there. His administrative team made daily rounds with the staff to show their appreciation, recognize the teams, and round for outcomes of what the staff needed support with to fulfill their jobs better. Did they need help with a process, equipment support, collaborative meetings, or any other need they wanted to bring up? By making consistent, daily connections, this CEO and his team were building relationships, trust, and dialogue to allow the employees to help steer the ship. This administrative team was also setting an example for all the other leaders in the organization to follow—directors, managers, supervisors, coordinators, and leads.

I have always been a firm believer that simple things make the most significant difference, and when people get to know each other, they want to help. The more we help each other, the more team spirit and trust we build. The more team spirit and trust we build, the faster the positivity machine starts to roll, picking up momentum and creating an exciting workplace where people are celebrated, appreciated, and listened to. This is the power of relationships, which should be at the heart and essence of everything we do as leaders, creating positive relationships with our staff, employees, physicians, and communities.

These connections need to be purposeful and consistent. Mark your calendar for rounding for outcomes, one-on-one employee conversations, thank you cards, recognitions, and communication. A friend once told me, "We are as free as the birds, though we often don't recognize it," and I had a CEO tell our entire team, "Remember, employees are volunteers. Sure, they get paid to do their work, but ultimately, they are free to choose where they work and can turn in their resignation at a moment's notice." I have never forgotten those words of advice. Everyone who shows up for work, for the call of duty in healthcare, or any field, has done so willingly. They made a choice today to show up and work, and if we treat them right, engage them, support them, and listen to them, odds are they will continue to show up and complete the vital work that needs to be accomplished. This is highly purposeful, meaningful, and rewarding work. We owe it to our patients, physicians, and communities to build relationships with our employees, listen to them, and support them to help develop positive and sustainable cultures.

POSITIVELY PERSISTENT

"Positively Persistent" is a phrase I have coined during my time as a leader. Sometimes you have a dream, a vision, an initiative, or a goal that you genuinely believe in, yet the journey is ripe with obstacles, setbacks, and disappointments. I tell my employees and fellow leaders now that if you genuinely believe it is the right thing to do for our patients, our community, and each other, you must stay positively persistent in your pursuit of that quest. You are the only one who is going to feel as strongly about your initiative and help keep the idea alive. Without you and your pursuit, the dream dies.

So, if you believe it to be the right thing, do not let it go. Along the journey, there will be times when you need to back off or lay low and wait for the right timing. You will always need to be respectful of others' opinions and biases, listen to their concerns, and present ideas from a different perspective. I have been involved in many projects that, in the initial planning stages, were met with a solid "No, that's never going to happen," to eventually finding the right timing and a path to completion.

A point of illustration involved implementing in-house MRI in a critical access hospital.

MRI Project: During my first leadership position as the Director of Imaging at a critical access hospital, we served our patients by providing X-ray, CT, ultrasound, mammography, and MRI. Our MRI unit was a mobile unit available three days out of the week. The new section of the hospital had been constructed over the previous five years and stood as the most modern and beautiful critical access hospital in the area.

During the construction phase, the administrative team had built a shell that would one day, hopefully, house an in-house MRI unit. It wasn't even my idea, and in the complexities of the financial world, the project for an in-house MRI unit had been set aside as not possible due to low monthly volumes failing to meet the financial threshold for success.

I held this leadership position as the Director of Imaging for five years, and during those five years, I dreamed about finding a way to bring MRI in-house. At first, I would write proposals with volume projections and capital budget requests that were repeatedly denied. During our capital budget meetings, where leaders throughout the hospital gathered in a room to argue cases for their projects, in-house MRI became a running joke. In good humor, people would rib me about my crazy dream of bringing MRI in-house. At first, I felt a little defensive and would reply with something like, "You must conceptualize it before it can come to fruition." It's how all dreams manifest. This really got the team going, and they would let me have it in good fun. After a couple of years, I wouldn't even bring the concept up, and still, someone would say that I was going to take all the capital budget money with my MRI project. "Ha ha," I would joke back.

On the inside, I knew there must be a way. The community needed more accessibility to MRI exams. That's when I had a chance encounter with a 3D tomosynthesis mammography vendor. During the visit, she told me a story about how another critical access hospital had acquired a Murdock grant for $250,000 and paid to implement their 3D tomosynthesis unit in their hospital at half the cost. The MJ Murdock Charitable Trust is a nonprofit organization that has been helping communities since 1975 to improve the arts and culture, education, health, human services, and scientific research for the betterment of all. The organization has invested more than 1.1 billion dollars into nonprofits for various initiatives to help dreams come true and positively benefit communities.

This was a huge epiphany for me. If another critical access hospital could accomplish it, why couldn't we? I quickly went to work on a proposal for the administrative team. I researched, planned, and wrote the proposal with specific details on how the capital budget money would be acquired from the Murdock grant and how much our hospital would be responsible for—just half the cost. I envisioned the future, created the business proposal, submitted it to the administrative team, and then waited anxiously for their response. I was sure this was our ticket to in-house MRI.

The first meeting was with the CEO herself. I was asked to meet with her to review my in-house MRI business proposal. I remember walking to the meeting and thinking, *It's been four years since we first brought up the idea, and now after staying true to the dream, staying positively persistent, it was going to come to fruition.* I was so excited. In my mind, I remember planning a celebration with my team. My wife and I would certainly go out to dinner that night to celebrate the good news.

Then, sitting across the desk from the CEO in excited anticipation after some small talk about the weekend weather, the CEO said, "Scott, I know you've put a lot of work into this project, but I need you to stop. There just aren't any more grant monies out there, and we need to focus on other priorities."

My heart sank. This wasn't the meeting that I thought I was attending. My ego crept up. I wanted to protest, ask why, and explain, but I could tell by her expression that she was resolute in her decision. I respectfully reminded her about the other critical access hospital that had received $250,000 for their project, and again she told me that this project needed to be put to rest for now. I left the office a bit dejected and felt sorry for myself. All that time, commitment, and energy spent on the idea, the initiative, the dream, and the business proposal to get to the front door of the CEO of the company, only to be told there were no more grants out there. The project was killed before it ever got started.

For the next year, I laid low on the MRI project. At the capital budget meeting, my colleagues again ribbed me about the dream of an in-house MRI. I smiled and took the ribbing. What else could I do? And yet, I truly believed that if we went for it and reached out to the MJ Murdock Charitable Trust, we had a good chance of bringing the project to fruition. That's when it happened.

Almost a year to the day after my first meeting with the CEO, she invited me back for another discussion about my business proposal for an in-house MRI. Since then, I had also added the idea of 3D tomosynthesis for mammography, a technology that would revolutionize mammography by increasing sensitivity and specificity by more than forty percent. This advancement in technology would allow us to detect much smaller lesions at much earlier stages of their development and ultimately save lives.

At the meeting, the CEO explained that they had rethought the idea of in-house MRI and 3D tomosynthesis and wanted to meet my grant writer. I was ecstatic and immediately set up a meeting with the grant writer and my administrative team.

Three weeks later, everything was set as the administrative team and I waited in the executive board room. Five minutes past the meeting start time, I started to worry. I tried calling our grant writer. With no answer, I was forced to leave a message. Ten minutes past the start time, things started to feel a little awkward. After all, the administrative team had vital work to do, and wasting their time in a meeting that wasn't happening was not one of them. Fifteen minutes past the start time with still no grant writer, I thought to myself, *This is it: Almost to the finish line and it's all over before they even get a chance to meet her.*

I started to apologize and check to see if we could reschedule, but I saw the look of skepticism on the leaders' faces. You don't hold up an entire administrative team for fifteen minutes past the expected start time of a meeting and expect a good outcome.

Then, in the middle of the potential reschedule, she showed up. Her positive energy and sincere apology for getting stuck in construction in a no-cell zone won the administrative team over. And just like that, we were on to the presentation. By the end of the question-and-answer period, I could tell that she had won over the entire executive team. Our project would be endorsed. By a unanimous consensus, the project launched with planning, research, and timeline implementation.

Over the course of five years, with so many doubts, my own theory had been legitimized. Staying positively persistent, knowing when to back off and lay low at times, and always remaining respectful of others' opinions and biases had paid off in a big way. The in-house MRI was going to come to fruition after all this time, nearly five years of dreaming, planning, strategizing, and negotiating. However, I wasn't going to be a part of it, at least not at my current hospital.

Unexpectedly, the opportunity to serve in my community presented itself. I accepted the Director of Imaging position in my hometown. For the previous five years, I had been commuting to work, a thirty-mile drive that went through two other towns and took about an hour each way. I was thrilled to have the opportunity to take on a more extensive department and serve in my own community. It also meant getting back two additional hours per day by avoiding the commute. I felt blessed and lucky to have the opportunity to serve my community and spend more time with my family. Honestly, though, it was heart-wrenching to leave my position. I had fallen in love with the people I worked with and grieved deeply leaving my team. I felt better about leaving the team in good hands when one of my technologists stepped up to take over the director position. Believing in leaving things better than when I found them, I provided six weeks of notice and transition time to ensure that everything was in good shape before leaving.

In my new position, two things happened within the first month that reminded me that our hard work is not always rewarded on our timelines. For one of my first public assignments, I found myself leading the open house of our 3D tomosynthesis unit, a project I had worked so hard to campaign for and implement in my previous hospital. The entire region implementing tomosynthesis was a direct result of one of my mammography technologists at my last site asking to be sent to a 3D tomosynthesis conference. Once she returned, we started our grant initiative for 3D tomosynthesis and in-house MRI. The reading radiology group read for several hospitals and happened to read for our hospital and the one I would eventually end up transferring to. The lead radiologist wanted to ensure that the hospital in my neighborhood, their main hub, would be the first in the area to acquire 3D tomosynthesis. She went directly to the administrative team to gain financial support. An executive decision was made, and the hospital in my community—not the one where I had worked and initiated the idea—ended up getting 3D tomosynthesis first. Within three years, the entire Pacific Northwest would have 3D tomosynthesis. I attribute that to a dream my lead technologist had in a simple request to go to a conference to learn more about 3D tomosynthesis.

In my new role, I led the open house as the Director of Imaging and reaped the rewards of the work that had been completed at my previous hospital where the dream and idea manifested. I knew in my heart that we should all be thanking my lead technologist at my last facility for making a dream come true, a dream with a technological advantage of increasing sensitivity and specificity by over forty percent, ultimately detecting cancers much earlier than previously possible with 2D and saving countless lives.

One month after I started my new directorship, I received a call from the grant writer of my former workplace. She called to say that she knew how hard I had pushed for the grant for 3D tomosynthesis and in-house MRI and she wanted me to be the first to know that my previous hospital was receiving an MJ Murdock Charitable Trust grant for $500,000 to assist with the implementation of 3D tomosynthesis and in-house MRI. I nearly fell out of my chair. Dreams come true if you are willing to put in the work, stay positively persistent, and never let the dream fade; after all, no one will care as much about your dreams as you do. Stay positively persistent; if you can think it, see it, dream it, and are willing to work hard for it, you can make that dream come to fruition. There will be setbacks, doubt, and times when you feel like giving up, but if you stay true to your passions and have patience, I have learned that anything is possible.

THE THREE R'S

Recruiting, Re-Recruiting, Retention

Today, more than ever, recruiting, re-recruiting, and retention play a significant role in an organization's success. As a healthcare leader, I believe there are two questions employees, leaders, and physicians need to be able to answer to create sustainability and longevity: 1) Why do you want to serve the community you live in? 2) Why do you want to serve your organization? The first question is often easier to answer for employees with ties to the community in which they live. The second question can be harder to respond to if the company's mission, vision, and values are not followed, if employees are not supported, and if open communication and transparency do not exist. Too often communications fail, relationships falter, and connectedness to purpose goes unhighlighted. In these situations, we often see people leave in search of more meaningful and connected work.

Without a connection to meaning, purpose, and worthwhile work, a connectedness to the mission, vision, and values, and a purposeful effort to create working relationships that assume positive intent, organizations will struggle to recruit and retain employees or run the risk of disengaging them. This results in higher turnover, lower engagement, poor quality and safety outcomes, and poorer employee and patient experiences.

To recruit employees, especially in today's competitive and destabilized market, organizations must demonstrate their commitment to the community, employees, transparency, best practices, and consistency in carrying out the mission, vision, and values. Now more than ever, caregivers find themselves disillusioned with their regular job and seek greener pastures or at least more lucrative pay with traveling assignments.

Though becoming a traveler has its benefits in being more lucrative for the caregiver, it poses some serious concerns for organizations and communities. On one hand, there are serious investments and costs associated with hiring employees who work for traveling companies to the tune of two to three times a regular salary. Another financial risk involves charting and charging and how well the traveling employees are trained and oriented on capturing accurate charges; if not done correctly, organizations stand to lose thousands of dollars in potential revenue. On the other hand, there is the risk and concern around safety and quality. Imagine an operating room department where fifty percent of its employees are travelers. This scenario is loaded with potential problems—the loss of historical information, no history of relationships with the physicians and other staff, and a lesser understanding of protocols, policies, and procedures—all of which can lead to safety and quality issues. Ideally, organizations will find the right combination in this new healthcare setting to attract and retain talent for building a sustainable team, enabling the opportunity to implement best practices and pivot quickly to changing demands in the industry.

For sustainability, we need to ask a question. What do employees really want? Throughout my career, the three initiatives that rise to the top of employee engagement surveys every year involve improving communication, a sense of autonomy, and growth opportunities. When you think about it, it's pretty much what we all desire as humans: a positive flow of communication, the ability to make some decisions, and the opportunity to learn and grow from our experiences.

Throughout the pandemic, I believe leaders felt like they were communicating more than ever before as the situation changed, sometimes day to day in the beginning. Yet, the engagement surveys often demonstrated employee dissatisfaction with leadership communication.

Why was this? Well, for one, we were all isolated due to the pandemic. Meetings went virtual and email communication increased while townhalls and in-person meetings stopped altogether. The changes happened so quickly during the first part of the pandemic that the morning's information was outdated by the afternoon. One-way communication, though necessary at times, is not what employees desire; they want their voices heard, their ideas heard, and the "why" communicated back to them. They desire communication from top to bottom, bottom to top, and side to side to reach a higher level of cooperation and understanding for the entire organization.

To succeed, we as leaders need to communicate in many ways, including email, phone, huddles, department meetings, townhalls, and rounding. We also need to be willing to listen to our employees' needs, wants, and ideas for improvement and act on the ones we can. We all want to belong to something larger than ourselves. This nurturing environment will give employees an answer to their second question: Why do you want to work for this organization?

As a leader, every encounter you have with an employee is an opportunity to re-recruit. Take time to listen, engage, and show interest in their lives, concerns, and ideas. After all, employees are the most significant resources and assets to the organization; through them, extraordinary work will reach the patient for the best outcomes. I've never forgotten the words of my former CEO, the one who encouraged us to always remember that every employee is ultimately a volunteer, because people can always change their minds and choose to work for a different organization or in a different community. I try to carry that idea into every interaction with employees. Please don't give them a reason to change their mind. Please treat them with compassion, respect, and gratitude for choosing your organization and community to serve.

ROUNDING AND REVIEWS

Employees are our greatest assets, and as leaders, it is our job to create cultures and environments where employees can thrive to their greatest potential. This is beneficial not only for the individual, but also for the patients, the organization, and the community. When we take this approach, we are no longer living in a world of winners and losers; we are living in a world of kindness and compassion where it is possible to create supporting cultures where all can thrive. Everyone has unique talents and skills. It is our job as leaders to take each employee from where they are and provide learning opportunities, remove barriers, and create cultures of trust for the employee's ultimate success. Their success is our success, so celebrate the good stuff, build momentum, and watch your employees, departments, and organizations thrive.

Informal rounding and formal rounding are two important ways to form bonds, foster relationships, and discover what needs to be accomplished or improved. I firmly believe that both rounding styles play a significant role in building teams and creating cultures. One without the other, however, will fail to bring out the full potential of your employees.

Informal Rounding: This type of rounding is fun, helps foster and build relationships, and consequently helps build trust. This is getting to the essence of our shared experiences as human beings. Sharing stories, pictures, and aspects of our lives is fun and interesting, helps spark imagination, and informs us of things we might want to try. A colleague and I started running after work on occasion, and during those runs, I learned about his experiences with marathons. He had qualified and run the Boston Marathon three times. Intrigued by such a feat—as I hadn't run more than four or five miles at the time—I started inquiring about how one trains for a marathon, what the experience is like, and wondering if I could run that far. One year later, I ran my first marathon.

By sharing stories, we expand our knowledge and curiosity. New worlds and possibilities open to us—adventures we previously may have never thought possible.

Formal Rounding, or rounding for outcomes, is a quest to uncover what we don't know. With specific and focused questions, we can find obstacles preventing our employees from doing their best work, discover what their professional aspirations are, and uncover whom they might recognize for doing a great job. We can reveal how collaboration is going with other departments along with an entire host of additional valuable information—information that will allow us as leaders to support our employees and teams.

Fostering questions may look something like this: "What's working well today?" "Any equipment or supplies you need?" "Anyone we should recognize today?" "Any process improvement ideas?" and "How is our collaboration with other departments?"

By focusing on specific questions, we can uncover specific answers. Once you have gleaned information from your crew, ask yourself: What did you learn? What actions do you need to take as a result? One of the most discouraging things for employees is speaking up without follow-up action. It is our job as leaders to follow up with an action plan or provide the communication as to why we cannot take action at that time. Sometimes we want to implement an action, initiative, or project but the timing doesn't align. In these instances, I encourage myself and my teams to stay positively persistent in pursuing our goals, aspirations, initiatives, and dreams. If the answer is no today, that does not mean the answer will be no in the future.

As leaders, there are tasks and work we need to do at our desks. This is a fact of the job. However, we will not learn what is happening in our departments at our desks. We will not learn what questions our employees have, what ideas they have, what frustrations they have, and we will not be able to make connections, build relationships, and create pathways of trust at our desks.

By purposefully planning our day, we can accomplish our desk work and take time to round, informally and formally, and find out what is happening at the front line. By doing this, we demonstrate to our employees that we believe the best ideas come from frontline staff; that our relationships and trust building are essential; and that by positively collaborating, we can build robust cultures, purposeful strategies, and teams, departments, and organizations that exude excellence. By connecting to mission, vision, and values, holding steadfast to consistency, and aligning our initiatives around patients, employees, and physicians, we will create teams, departments, and organizations that are resilient in leading the way to what right looks like.

So, get out there and find out what you don't know. I promise you that it will be worth the effort. By doing so, you will ultimately be supporting the community.

Reviews: Organizations may conduct reviews at different times. Most common are quarterly or annual reviews. Being purposeful and consistent with your review process will enable you to make connections, build relationships, uncover information, and provide a formal opportunity to re-recruit your employees. The costs of turnover (costs of hiring + training + severance or bonus package + loss of historical information + loss of productivity + increased burnout of remaining staff filling in + loss of personal connections and relationships) generally equate currently to six to nine months of that employee's salary. In today's market, with the staff shortage, we can also factor in traveling expenses, which are two to three times the average staff salary. If we want to take it a step further, we need to factor in the loss of knowledge and experience and the loss of connections between employees and physicians who had previously established trust. This can and will most likely result in a loss of consistency in safety and quality. When you get teams of people unfamiliar with each other working side by side, you run the risk of communication breakdown, misunderstanding of processes or protocol, and lack of organizational history, all of which can lead to poor outcomes and potential harm to patients.

Retention and re-recruiting are key to consistency and sustainability, so don't skip this step of formal rounding in the form of monthly, quarterly, and annual connections and reviews. This is your opportunity to connect with your employee formally; manage and recognize all their successes; understand what their career aspirations and dreams are; and connect their role to the overall mission, vision, and values of the organization and how that positively impacts the department, organization, and the community. Take time on your formal reviews; I recommend allotting an hour for each annual review. If you have a large team, you may consider breaking the reviews up by quarters of the year. Though this is time-consuming, it is one of the most significant investments you will make to help build and sustain culture.

The review process highlighted here is not a traditional review highlighting if the employee is doing a "good" or "bad" job. We need to eliminate those types of biased words from our leadership perspective and instead look at the formal review as an opportunity to see how we as leaders can support them on their career paths and journeys toward success. Their success is our success. Any types of disciplinary action or concerns should be addressed immediately—I recommend not waiting or utilizing the formal review as a time to point out mistakes, errors, or corrections the employee needs to make; this will only discourage and disengage the employee. Instead, hold yourself accountable for coaching in the moment. If there is a mistake, an error, or disciplinary action that needs to be addressed, address it immediately. Do not look the other way or wait in hopes that the behavior will self-correct. If you do, you are not holding yourself accountable as a leader and are not keeping your commitments to your employees; as a great coach once told me, "Remember, coaching is caring."

If you care about the employee, the department, the organization, and the community, you will address things as they come up with compassion and respect.

By doing this, you will avoid situations spinning out of control and growing larger than they need to.

Sometimes we assume the employee knows they are doing something outside the mission, vision, values, and standards of excellence. Don't make this mistake. Assume nothing and address the issue as a coach. If the pattern or behavior persists, you may have to involve your human resource partners to address the issue more formally. However, initially assume positive intent and give your employees the chance to self-correct; it is the compassionate thing to do and the action that will build the most trust. Ultimately, once the employee understands the expectations, it is their choice to do the right thing or not. As a leader, once you make the expectations visible, it gets harder and harder to not do the right thing.

THE FOUR C'S AND THEN SOME

Compassion, Collaboration, Creativity, Collective Teamwork, Clarity, Communication, Customer Service, Service Recovery

Compassion: Being present and purposefully trying to see life from another's perspective will help us be more compassionate, whether that other person is a patient, a family member, a colleague, or a physician. Compassion allows us to help others heal both emotionally and physically. A commitment to compassion will enable us to step outside ourselves and help others. This is why we were all drawn to healthcare in the first place, to do meaningful work that makes a difference in another's life. This focus will help us build relationships and combat burnout.

Collaboration: By collaborating with others, we align with our mission, vision, and values to help our initiatives, goals, and dreams come to fruition. We unleash a vast array of possibilities by engaging each other's ideas and being open to new perspectives. This collaboration has the energy to change our course for the better and to reach our true potential as individuals, departments, organizations, and communities.

Creativity: Engaging in our imagination allows us to think creatively and take on challenges with new perspectives and an open mindset. Challenging the norms will allow us to unlock new solutions for today's and tomorrow's problems. In the current complexities of healthcare, the solutions that worked in the past may not work in today's environment. By allowing others to add their creativity to the mix, we'll have an entire organization looking for new solutions and answers to the obstacles that arise. So often, the best ideas come from frontline staff; don't hesitate to give your employees a voice to unlock this potential for the best outcomes.

Collective Teamwork: Much like collaboration, but with a purpose toward a specific outcome. Collective teamwork believes that all voices and ideas should be heard and thoughtfully discussed to identify the best course of action. By utilizing collective teamwork, you engage your team in creating a safe culture where people are not afraid to speak up and share their ideas, opinions, concerns, and solutions.

Clarity: As leaders, we need to be clear with our teams on our communication by defining clarity of roles, goals, expectations, best practices, and how our work and initiative impact the organization from a strategic and mission-driven perspective. By connecting each position with the organization's overall mission and strategic vision, we tie purpose and meaning to our employees' work and how it positively impacts the organization and the community.

Communication: Communication must be transparent and distributed in many forms; don't make the mistake of thinking an email will reach all of your employees. Send emails, hold huddles, round, and hold department meetings, townhalls, and community events to ensure your message is delivered and received. Creating forums that provide a feedback loop where clarifying questions can be asked will allow us to build trust, relationships, and a foundation for creating centers of excellence.

Customer Service: Patients are why we are all here. Without patients, we can all pack up and go home. Committing to our patients every time we treat them with compassion and respect, meeting them where they are, explaining and answering questions, and following through with action that matches our words will build essential relationships with our patients to get them on the road to recovery. Being in the moment and present with our patients, calling them by their names, introducing ourselves, and taking the time to explain and answer questions will help build rapport, ease fears and anxieties, and provide the opportunity for the best outcomes.

Service Recovery: Sometimes, things don't always go as planned. For example, a patient may be upset about their bill and doesn't understand their co-pay or why a specific portion of the exam or procedure was not covered. These are some of the best moments to engage in compassion, respect, and understanding by stepping outside ourselves and seeing it through our patient's eyes. If we make a mistake or error, we first need to report this in our Safety Alert System and then uncover what action we need to take to make it right with our patient and their family. We must admit when something did not go as planned and let them know how we are correcting our practice so the error or mistake does not reach another patient. Though it may not help our current patient and their complaint, my experience in these conversations has unequivocally demonstrated that people are grateful when we are open, honest, and humble with them and let them know that their experience is going to ensure it doesn't happen to other people.

If it is a billing issue, patients often do not understand their co-insurances and co-pays, or they do not have the funds to meet their deductibles. These are times when you can engage your financial counselors to help with discounted or no interest rate payments, financial assistance, or other assistance that your organization or community can support. One of my organizations had a program set up for anyone who did not have insurance and could not afford a mammogram. Those patients could call and mention our program, and with no questions asked, we would schedule them for their appointment and set up the payments with our foundation. This program was supported by donations from our annual Pink Tea community event established for this specific reason. What a great opportunity and contribution to the community for donors to make a difference in another's life. Does your organization have a program like this? If not, consider starting one or proposing the idea to a superior.

ONBOARDING

The importance of onboarding cannot be overstated. This is our opportunity to connect our employees to our mission, vision, and values; clarify their roles and how they tie into the overall strategic vision of the organization; set clear expectations for our standards of behavior; and introduce policies, procedures, and critical pieces of knowledge to set the employee or leader up for success.

Onboarding should take place on an organizational and departmental level where the employee is introduced to the tools to perform their job, access necessary resources, and orient on how to locate information and people. The most successful organizations will organize a welcoming committee for the first day, plan a lunch tour, and assign a mentor to help guide the new employee or leader.

These mentorships can last a few weeks to many, depending on whether the employee is a seasoned professional or just starting their careers. Regardless, our recommendation is a minimum of a four-week mentorship program to help align the new employee to the organization's standards, practices, and people, as well as the mission, vision, and values. More investment upfront will increase the probability of engagement, long-term employment, and a connection to the organization's higher purpose. *Invest* in your employees; build positive cultures and vital strategic initiatives covering the healthcare pillars of *people, service, quality, finance,* and *growth;* and watch this manifest into best practices and success for your people, organization, and community.

OPERATIONS

We can dig into processes now that we have established our culture. First, we have found that our people are our greatest asset. Second, turnover is incredibly costly to an organization in many ways, including costs of recruiting and training, loss of consistency, loss of historical information, loss of safety, and loss of quality. To have streamlined operations, we need a robust, engaged staff connected to mission, vision, and values and fully oriented and trained in their positions. As leaders, it is our responsibility to ensure these things are taking place before we ever think of streamlining operations.

Reviewing operations, not all areas will generate revenue or make a profit. Some areas may lose money and be justifiable in lining up with the community needs assessment. If operations profit and losses balance out in the end, we may be able to justify areas of loss in order to provide the necessary care our community needs.

As leaders, there are a few cost areas we can help influence into positive outcomes: supplies and salaries.

With supplies, we can work with our value analysis teams, procurement departments, and vendors to help identify cost savings for supplies, equipment, and contracts. We must negotiate these areas to procure the best value for our organization. In most business deals, there is room for negotiation and a better price if we are willing to push the issue. With today's inflated costs, we must remain steadfast in pursuing the best prices to stay financially firm.

Salaries and FTE counts are within our control, though this is a complicated area. As organizations, focusing on productivity, reducing FTE, and implementing low census to send people home during downtime is easy. However, I have never favored low census of staff unless it is on a volunteer basis. After all, everyone has budgeted their life based on their salary, and it is dissatisfying to be forced to leave work early. Having staff create lists of what is appropriate to work on during downtime is a great way to add value to the organization. As for FTE count, we need to be leery of striving for one hundred percent productivity while running the staff too lean. This strategy generally results in increased overtime when staff call out or are on extended leave, increased burnout, and a higher turnover rate. Once this occurs, the organization ends up paying two to three times the amount in recruitment and traveler expenses, which is unsustainable in the long run.

A better strategy for operations is to focus on retention programs, engagement work, and building relationships with the staff. These approaches will ultimately save money in the long run, build solid and sustainable teams, and avoid unnecessary expenses.

Streamlining operations involves asking questions, conducting research, and discovering the best practice for a particular area. Collaborating with other hospitals, researching professional journals and organizations, and implementing those practices will help align recommended best practices and outcomes.

The good news is that we do not have to reinvent the wheel with best practices. Though these tend to change over time, we have information at our fingertips these days, and almost instantaneous resources to uncover the recommendation for a specific best practice. We can create momentum, excitement, and progress toward improvement and excellence by engaging our teams and allowing them to be part of the discovery process.

For new leaders, it's paramount that they receive the support they need from IT, finance, and leadership to ensure that they have an understanding of the systems, expectations, and financial statements to run their department effectively. So often, it's assumed that new leaders automatically know their department's financial programs, statements, and cost centers.

If this is not already part of your orientation process, I highly recommend adding it to your onboarding process for new leaders in order to set them up for success in understanding the financial workings of their departments.

Though there have been numerous books written on operational excellence from a financial perspective, my philosophy remains solid that if you support your employees, build the culture, and align with the mission, vision, and values by connecting to purpose and meaning, all other areas will more easily fall into place with purposeful attention.

NET RETURN

Invest in people + build a culture based on mission, vision, and values + implement strategies based on the five pillars: people, service, quality, finance, and growth + continuous process improvement = best outcomes. What we put into something is what we will get out of something, and that "something" is all about people.

YOU NEED TO FIRE THEM

Three times in my career, I have been approached out of the blue and told that I needed to fire someone. Three times, in each of those instances, I have asked for clarity, grace, and time to coach the person. I have yet to fire someone under these circumstances.

Case One

No more than a day after I assumed my first leadership role as Director of Imaging, I was approached by my administrative team that I needed to fire the department secretary. Caught off guard, I inquired why this information was not disclosed during the interview process. In fact, the secretary had been on the hiring committee and seemed nice, compassionate, and engaged. The crux of the problem, I was to learn, was that the physician group was fed up with dealing with her; she was a bad apple and had to go. I inquired further about the main source of the physician's complaint. After all, this secretary was quite friendly in manner and speech. I couldn't imagine her being rude or hard to get along with. The problem, I learned, was that when the physicians wanted to run a same-day CT exam as an add-on study, the secretary always told them the department could not accommodate their patient, no exceptions. The county our hospital served was one of the largest in all of the state with so many of our patients traveling over an hour to attend a doctor's visit. Hearing the complaint, I understood the physician's frustration, let alone the inconvenience to the patient in time wasted and extra expense. Hearing the problem, I told the administration that I would speak with the secretary and make clear our expectations of being able to add on cases for the physician group.

In my office, I asked the secretary why the answer was always no to the physician group when they wanted to add a CT patient onto the current day's schedule. She calmly told me that the last director insisted that the patients needed a full prep the night before and no routine exams were to be added on the day of. When I heard this, I clearly understood that the secretary was not being obstinate but simply following the instructions of her previous boss. I then told the secretary that I wanted her to add on any patient that the physician group wanted to add on; we would simply use the quick prep for oral contrast and scan the patient that day. We'd be saving them time and money by not having to come back another day, and we would get the results faster for the patient and the physician. The secretary was elated that she would now be able to say yes to the physician group. Ironically, over the next year, our secretary received great praise and recognition from the physician group and was touted as the best patient advocate by the group. This was a great lesson to me; things aren't always what they seem, and unless you as a leader are willing to do your own investigation, seek your own clarity, and set your own expectations with your employees, you may end up missing out on some great wins. In this case, our secretary went from being despised and seen as a roadblock to one of the most praised individuals of our department. She was allowed to make things happen and help people in the moment, giving her great satisfaction and meaning in her work.

Case Two

It was the first time I had hired an ultrasonographer from California. She was right out of school and eager to kick-start her career. Pleasant in demeanor, consistent in her work, and compassionate about her profession and patients, she fit right in. She'd been working for us just over a year when the lead radiologist came into my office and said I needed to fire my newest ultrasonographer.

"Fire her?" I said, perplexed, as I had not heard any negative reviews about this person.

The radiologist insisted that her work was just not up to par with the other technologists and the other radiologists had lost faith and confidence in her work. Yes indeed, in their opinions, I needed to fire her.

I was taken aback and told my lead radiologist that I was not about to fire my newest technologist, as this was the first I was hearing there were any issues with her work. I told the lead radiologist that I would talk to her and explain where she currently was, that her school had left out some important aspects of her training, blind spots that she needed to correct, and that we would need to dedicate the next three months to getting her work up to par with the other ultrasonographers and earn back the faith and trust of the radiologists.

In all my years of leadership, I had never felt so certain that I would sooner sacrifice my own job for the cause than fire her. We met in my office, and I explained to her that there was a gap in her training, that the radiologists were questioning her skills, and that I needed her to work harder to learn, grow, and improve her skills. I promised her that if she did these things, it was all going to work out and that I and the ultrasound team would support her in her studies, review, and critiques of her work. She agreed with tears in her eyes and went to work learning the blind spots that her school had left lacking.

Fast-forward a year, two years, five years later, and our newest ultrasonographer, hired right out of school from California, had not only learned her blind spots, earned the respect of the radiologists and fellow colleagues, but had become one of our best ultrasonographers in the entire organization. This was another great lesson: Never underestimate what people are capable of achieving given the right circumstances, coaching, and adequate time to improve their knowledge, skills, and care.

Had I not questioned the radiologists and just fired my newest hire on their wishes, we all would have missed out on a fantastic technologist and an amazing person. Give people the right chance and dare them to prove you wrong, and you just might find that something extraordinary happens.

Case Three

The day before the Director of Patient Access was let go, I was called in to the administrative office. There I was asked by the CEO and Director of Human Resources if I would act as Interim Director of Ancillary Services. Hesitating at first, I struggled to say no, as I always wanted to help the organization out when I could. As long as it was only on an interim basis until they found a permanent hire, I was okay with the role. Little did I know that the interim role would last for over four years.

Upon accepting the role, I was then informed that they thought I should fire the coordinator who worked directly under the director who was just let go. This request sounded familiar to me. I had been in this situation before, and I knew what to say. I listened to their concerns about the coordinator. There was fear that the coordinator was just like the director, two peas in a pod, so to speak, and that if I didn't fire her, I would achieve little to no success with the team. I told them I understood their fears and requested they give me some time to work with the coordinator, set my own clear expectations, and provide coaching and support before we made a final decision. Reluctantly, the administrative team agreed to give it a try. What I soon learned was that, just as my secretary at my previous organization was following the guidance of her former leader, so too was this coordinator following the lead of her boss even though deep down she wanted to do things differently. We were both relieved to learn that we had similar healthcare philosophies, believed in servant leadership and that the best ideas come from frontline staff, and wanted to install a professionalism in the Patient Access Crew, the gatekeepers of the hospital, that had been lacking under the previous leadership.

Within a couple of months, I was called to a meeting with the administrative team. They told me whatever I was doing with the coordinator was working wonders. The team was acting more professionally, patient satisfaction was up, and turnover was down in that department. I received the compliment humbly and told them that the coordinator was previously acting on behalf of her boss for fear of retaliation and that she was relieved she could now include the staff in more of the decision making, process improvements, and building up of the overall culture. In retrospect, the only thing I did was set clear expectations, provide support when needed, and help remove barriers so that this particular coordinator and her team could thrive. And thrive they did. The coordinator was the only one certified in both the American Association of Healthcare Administrative Management (AAHAM) and National Association of Healthcare Access Management (NAHAM). She inspired many others to achieve their certifications and provide a culture of learning and educational growth opportunities for herself and her team.

Once again, I was reminded that holding others accountable without providing coaching and support is cruelty. Before we pass judgment or activate corrective action plans, we as leaders must first ask ourselves if we have provided adequate training, orientation, support, clear expectations, and ongoing coaching sessions to help guide our employees and leaders to alignment with our mission, vision, and values. If we have exhausted all of these avenues and still things are not falling in alignment, then and only then do we need to start down the path of corrective action. So many times we jump ahead in the process, failing to give our employees, future leaders, and current ones the necessary tools, support, and coaching to really thrive in an ever-changing environment. We owe that much to ourselves, our teams, our organizations, and our communities.

NEVER JUDGE A TORTOISE BY ITS START

I am making an assumption here when I ask, "Have you ever heard the story of the tortoise and the hare?"

Each year, in our imaging departments, we have radiology students that conduct semester-long clinical rotations. It's a great way for us to remember the things that we have forgotten and to groom potential new hires.

Every once in a while, a student will come along that makes me wonder why they chose radiology. This one particular student—let's call her Grace—had been with us for more than two months, hadn't taken an X-ray, and was just hanging back observing everything, apparently too shell-shocked to even help out with little things like setting the brake on a wheelchair. I spoke with my team about my concerns, and they all agreed. I began to wonder if Grace had chosen the wrong career field and if I should reach out to her clinical instructor. That's when the magic happened.

Grace and one of our senior technologists—let's call her Gwen—were working together. Gwen was taking the X-rays, and Grace was observing as normal. Then Gwen, a senior tech with over twenty years of experience, made a simple mistake—a rookie mistake, really—and made a joke about herself in front of Grace to lighten the mood. Whatever and however it was said, from that moment on, Grace let go of her apprehension, her holding back, and started taking the lead on exams. She charged ahead, completing her competencies in short order, and by the end of her four-month rotation, we had her not only doing every X-ray exam imaginable, but she was also competently learning CT.

At the end of her four-month rotation, I pulled Grace into my office and shared with her my concerns when she'd first come to our department. I was honest that I originally thought she had made a mistake on her career choice and wondered how I should break the news to her and her instructor. And now, four months later, I told her that she looked like a seasoned technologist, and I would hire her on the spot. Little did I know that over ten years later, I would be working at a much larger facility where we were installing the newest CT unit GE had to offer, and lo and behold, who was our CT applications engineer? Grace!

This was a huge lesson to myself as a new leader and to our entire team: Never assume that just because a new student or employee starts off slow that they will remain there. It just so happens that some of them will go on to become your greatest employees, continuing to learn, grow, and take on new responsibilities as the opportunities present themselves. Creating a safe space for students and employees to thrive is the only way to help them actualize their full potential.

BOB
Making a Difference

Remember when I said it's the little things that can sometimes make the biggest difference? Bob is one of our transporters in radiology and an amazing human being. One day during a meeting, Bob shared a story with me about his morning. He told me that almost every day someone he is helping transport to the radiology department makes a lasting impression on him and inspires him in his own life. Usually, he said, it comes closer to the end of his ten-hour shift, but on this particular day, it came in the morning.

He was transporting a female patient in her mid-fifties back to her room when she starting complaining about a surgeon. Bob was surprised, as this particular surgeon she was complaining about was one patients generally raved about. Bob asked her why she was so upset. She replied indignantly, "Well, just look at what he did to my hair. I used to have such beautiful hair, now look at it." Back in the room, her husband was going on about how beautiful she still looked and what if she just shaved it completely. It would eventually grow back. The patient was having none of it and didn't want to hear another word.

Bob's next patient for transport happened to have had the same surgeon work on her. At thirty-five years of age, she had decided to completely shave her head. Bob commented on her decision to shave her entire head, and she replied quite enthusiastically, "It's only hair. After all, it will grow back."

After dropping his second patient off, Bob headed back to his first patient's room and shared with her the young lady's attitude about her hair and how it was no big deal, that it would grow back given enough time. The first patient smiled, taking the information in and said, "Huh." And then said, "Thank you for that. You're right, it is only hair, after all, and it will grow back." The patient was grateful for Bob taking the extra time to come back and share the story, and the husband was grateful for a second opinion that his wife was still beautiful with or without hair.

Now this story could have gone another way if the patient hadn't received the message, but the fact that Bob cared enough to try and help brighten another's day by sharing another perspective ... Well, he helped change the course of her outlook and helped relieve some of her suffering just by taking the time to share a story. That's the good stuff! Those little things make huge differences in others' lives.

What opportunities do you have to make a difference in another's life? Do you take advantage of those opportunities? Or let them slip through the cracks in the day?

It's up to you now. Go forth, lead as a servant, celebrate the little things, and see how the magic of human connection and compassion can heal our patients, ourselves, and our communities.

NURSE ERIN

Making a Difference

Sixteen years. That's the amount of time that would go by before I wrote the letter. Life moves at the blink of an eye. Sixteen years to say thank you. Thank you for caring for us, my wife, and our child. Thank you for caring so much and knowing how to ease our fears.

We didn't need a coach. It was our third birth, and we knew the techniques very well. "Hee-Hee-Hoo, Hee-Hee-Hoo" was taught back then, a breathing technique when the contractions began. With our firstborn, our son came out posterior with the cord wrapped around his neck. The doctor said, "I've got a floppy one here." Code to the nursing staff that our son was not breathing.

"Is the baby all right?" my wife asked repeatedly. Fearing the worst and not knowing, I repeated to my wife that the baby was all right, though my words sounded false to my ears.

Our son's Apgar score was a four. The Apgar score is a method to determine a baby's health at birth by assigning a score of zero to ten for five categories: appearance (skin color), pulse (heart rate), grimace response (reflexes), activity (muscle tone), and respiration (breathing rate and effort). A baby in good health scores a seven or above on the Apgar score.

While I reassured my wife that the baby was okay, the nurses and physician quickly went to work on our son, providing oxygen and working his muscles to life. Within minutes—which seemed like an eternity as I felt our dreams slipping away—our son came to life. My wife, now desperate in her question, repeated, "Is the baby okay?" As the doctor worked on my wife, he reassured her that he wouldn't be here if the baby wasn't alright. "Here" meant at the foot of the bed stitching my wife up as he joked about how our son looked like a boxer.

As I glanced over to where the nurses were treating our son, Joshua, all nine and a half pounds of him, I wondered what I was staring at. The purplish creature, a shade of color I had never quite seen before or since, raised its head and turned toward us. *My god,* I heard my mind's voice say, *we've given birth to an alien.* It took another five minutes of circulation to pump the purplish hue from his skin and for us to recognize him as a newly born human. As for our son being able to raise his head at birth, we hypothesized that my wife had so much amniotic fluid that our son could do backflips in the womb. He was at least a week beyond his due date, maybe more since he came out dry, enabling him to develop unusual neck strength. Our doctor and nurses were terrific at remaining calm, easing our fears, and caring for our son.

The birth of our second child—our daughter Olivia—was also a terrifying experience. Our nurse, realizing my wife was experiencing an extreme amount of anxiety leading up to the delivery—most likely post-traumatic stress disorder (PTSD) from our first birthing experience—asked the doctor if she could administer my wife a mild narcotic to ease her anxiety.

We listened as our doctor and nurse had a quiet side conversation about the matter, and we couldn't help but overhear that the doctor was somewhat reluctant to administer the narcotic if the birth was near. As he explained, it was our choice to have the narcotic administered, though we needed to understand that there were risks involved. One of the most concerning risks was that if they administered the narcotic and the baby was born within thirty minutes of administration, it could potentially damage the baby's lungs and complicate breathing.

After some discussion and reasonable assurance from our physician that it didn't appear my wife would give birth in the next thirty minutes, we decided to have the narcotic administered. Immediately, the medication calmed my wife's anxieties, and she relaxed and dozed off for brief moments. And then it happened. The nurse called our doctor back within fifteen minutes of administering the narcotic. My wife was in full-on labor. As our doctor entered the room, he said, "I'm worried about the baby." Again, we felt our world starting to crash around us. Both grandmothers, who had hoped to be bedside during the birth, remained in the waiting area as we found ourselves in a situation where the doctor and nursing team were going into rescue mode to counteract the narcotic as soon as our daughter was born to save her lungs and quite possibly her life. Fortunately, from the quick action of our doctor and nursing team, our daughter survived and developed a healthy set of lungs.

When our third child, Rosalind, was born, the birthing process was smooth sailing. My wife went into labor, and our baby girl was born less than ten minutes later. Our doctor handed me a pair of forceps, and I cut the umbilical cord—something I hadn't had the opportunity to perform during the births of our first two children.

The doctor handed our baby girl to my wife, congratulated us, and left the room. We began to rejoice, tears of joy, that we were blessed with a healthy baby and, this time, no complications. Then, something quickly went wrong. Our nurse called the doctor back into the room. Our daughter wasn't breathing correctly; something worried them that her lungs had not fully developed. The physician whisked our daughter out of the room. At this time, we had two nurses in the room: one whose name I don't remember, and the other, Nurse Erin.

Panicked, my wife asked what I was doing there and told me to check on the baby. I rushed out the door to the next room. The doctor and two other nurses had our baby in an incubator. They appeared to be assessing her breathing and checking her pulse. From the birthing room, I could hear my wife, in a raised voice, say, "Is the baby okay?" Once again, I found myself caught in the space of uncertainty and wanting to reassure my wife that the baby was okay, that everything was okay and would be okay. And yet, the most sinking, dreadful feeling overcame me as I studied the worried looks on our doctor's and nurses' faces.

I returned to the birthing room to report to my wife, and that's when it happened. Nurse Erin was pushing on my wife's abdomen, massaging the uterus back into position, and it appeared my wife was hemorrhaging. My head felt light at the sight of so much blood.

"Is this normal?" I heard my wife ask Nurse Erin as I came to her side. My wife glanced up at me, pure fear in her eyes.

Nurse Erin said calmly and with reassurance, "We don't like it when this happens, but we know what to do."

Medication was administered to counteract the bleeding as Nurse Erin continued to massage my wife's abdomen, working the uterus back into place. A mother's instinct to protect her children is much more powerful than her concern for her own well-being.

"What are you doing here?" my wife asked. "Go check on the baby." Feeling my worlds torn apart, wanting to save my wife and our baby and feeling completely helpless, I imagined the worst-case scenarios. What if I lost both of them? I ran back across the hallway to check on our baby. The doctor informed me that our daughter was having trouble breathing. They believed her lungs hadn't formed properly, and they would have to fly her to Sacred Heart Medical Center in Spokane, Washington. He said that there was only room for the baby and the crew on the helicopter, and that other family or I would have to make the ninety-minute drive to the hospital.

As soon as I entered the room, my wife knew something was wrong.

"What's wrong with the baby?"

I repeated the information from our doctor.

Without saying a word, my wife started to get out of the birthing bed.

"What are you doing?" the other nurse asked.

"I'm going with my daughter on the helicopter. They're not taking my baby without me," my wife proclaimed. There was desperation and sheer determination in her voice as she pushed past her pain and stood.

“She needs to see her baby,” Nurse Erin said calmly and with authority.

The other nurse protested, saying my wife was in no condition to get out of bed with her bleeding.

Again, Nurse Erin stated calmly and as a matter of fact, “She needs to see her baby,” as she prepared a wheelchair with chucks placed on the seat to soak up the blood.

The three of us—my wife, Nurse Erin, and I—went across the hallway. I positioned the wheelchair in front of the window so my wife could see our daughter tucked under the incubator. Nurse Erin went into the room to speak to the doctor. There was a brief conversation, glances back toward us, and then Nurse Erin gently retrieved our daughter from the incubator and brought her to my wife.

The rest of the story? Our daughter started to breathe normally for unknown reasons, possibly just the right amount of time for her lungs to fully form. The doctor checked her lungs, cleared her, and canceled the Life Flight helicopter. My wife’s bleeding came under control, and we later celebrated in our room with a candlelight dinner of steak, mashed potatoes, and veggies, followed by chocolate cake and ice cream while our daughter, Rosalind, slept peacefully.

It was indeed the most frightened I have been in all my life, the possibility of losing both my daughter and my wife in that moment.

And still, it took me sixteen years to express my gratitude and tell Nurse Erin what a difference she made at that moment.

I'd been teaching customer service classes in our hospital for years. As a storyteller, I would often lead by telling the story of Nurse Erin and Customer Extraordinaire John to get to the heart of making a difference. One day, a nurse in my class who knew Nurse Erin suggested I should tell her. After all, I had been telling others how much she meant to our family for years, and how at that moment, she had made such a powerful and positive impact on our life. The nurse who suggested I reach out just happened to have Nurse Erin's new address; years prior, she had moved from the area. Later that night, as I sat down to write the letter to Nurse Erin, it dawned on me how rare it is for us as human beings to express our gratitude and appreciation. So often, we are quick to criticize, complain, or write a letter of discontent. How many of us truly express our gratitude to the right person? Sure, we often tell friends, family, and even strangers about the nice gesture someone else did for us, but we rarely say it to the person we most appreciate.

This became a powerful lesson for myself, my leaders, and our caregivers. The lesson is that the things you do daily in healthcare and life can profoundly and positively impact others beyond our knowledge or understanding. You will often not hear back from your patients on what a fantastic job you did, how you eased their fears, helped them stay calm, and helped them receive the care they needed.

By staying in the moment and doing the best we can to care for others, we have a profound impact on our patients and each other, giving us great purpose and adding meaning to the work we do each day. This level of care transcends differences in worldviews, politics, life perspectives, and biases to bring people together in a healthy way.

If you have someone who has recently made a difference in your life, or one like mine that made a difference years ago, and you have not told them, I encourage you to reach out now in some small way to let them know how their caring helped you and your loved ones get through a difficult time. These actions are beyond powerful and will perpetuate the fantastic work that goes on in healthcare daily. For it's the good stuff that inspires us to push through the complexities, frustrations, and negativity surrounding healthcare for a better tomorrow. If you allow yourself, you can be inspired by that idea of a better tomorrow and become an essential and invaluable piece of making a difference.

AFTERWORD

At the beginning of my career, when asked what my most significant successes were, I would answer the question with personal accomplishments like obtaining my associate and bachelor's degrees, or becoming certified in X-ray, CT, and MRI, and all the projects and process improvements we as a team were able to accomplish. It wasn't until later in my career that this answer changed dramatically. Somewhere along the line, it was no longer about my accomplishments, or even my departments or areas where I provided leadership oversight. Rather it was how I was able to help another person accomplish their dreams. Now, when asked the question about my most significant accomplishments, they always center around opportunities to help support, motivate, or maybe even inspire another person into action. It is truly about them and their successes. I am humbled when others are open to allowing me to help. After all, it is hard sometimes to ask for and accept help. As leaders, we have opportunities to help others and see their professional dreams come true by creating connections, opening opportunities, and providing support and encouragement. This is the greatest pleasure in my career: How can I make a difference in another's life, no matter how big or small? So often, it is the little things that make the most significant differences—a phone call to a school to help an employee get accepted, a reference letter or call for a promotion, an opportunity to learn a new skill, or a formal rounding for outcomes to understand how you can support the employee better.

Leadership is one of the most complex, challenging, and rewarding careers you will ever embark on. You have the opportunity to help influence change, help people grow professionally, make connections, and partake in work that is meaningful and important to the community.

However, leadership is not for everyone. And that's okay. While transitioning from one leadership position to another, I mentored an employee to take over the leadership position I'd be vacating. He'd be taking over the radiology department. At first, he wasn't sure about leadership but was strongly considering it. The lead radiologist encouraged him to apply and told him to try it for a few months to see if he liked it. When he told me this, I smiled and chuckled. I informed him that he probably wouldn't like it for at least a year. He looked shocked when I told him this. I explained what I meant:

Though you will enjoy many aspects of the job, you will lose sleep for at least a year, feel like you don't know what you're doing, and find yourself second-guessing your decisions.

In many of those first days and months, you will look back at your day and wonder what you accomplished—so much of leadership remains in the abstract and is hard to quantify in specific terms or accomplishments. As a leader, you will not know all the answers that come your way; it takes time to grow. In the first year, these questions made me panic even before they were asked and kept me up at night. What if something comes up that I don't know?

Over time, I learned while working as a team and collaborating on problems that we can identify the answer and, in most cases, quickly move into action for a solution.

After more than twenty years of healthcare experience, there are still questions that come up daily that I do not know. Sometimes the answer is identified in minutes, and other times it takes time and collaboration. But with effort and teamwork, we always find the solution. I sleep much better these days.

After two years, my friend decided that leadership was not for him, and he went back to scanning patients in MRI and CT. He is one of the best technologists I have ever had the privilege to coach, mentor, and work alongside; he is a fantastic person and still an influential, informal leader. He helps make and contribute to critical daily decisions to provide excellent service to patients, the organization, and the community.

In my first year of leadership, I had a fellow leader say, "If you want to work in healthcare, there will always be important work to accomplish. It just might not be the current role you're in right now."

Serving others in healthcare has been a gift that elevates me beyond myself, my ego, and my biases to a place where I can help others. To me, healthcare is the gift that rises above differences, biases, prejudices, and preconceived notions to do our best work and have some of our best experiences. The people I have met in healthcare have been some of the best people I have ever had the privilege to meet and work alongside. For that, I am forever thankful.

And now I ask, what will your story be? And how can I help?

Sincerely,
Scott Nelson

ACKNOWLEDGMENTS

The publication of *Higher Ground* has been a collaborative effort with special thanks and recognition first and foremost to my wife, Lisa Marie, for all her support, encouragement, and feedback. Secondly, I'd like to thank Rebecca Dehlin, lead beta reader, as well as all the professionals who brought this book to life in the editing, design, and launch phases: Joel Pitney (Founder of Launch My Book), Sayde Walker (Managing Director), Stephen Parkin (Managing Editor), Pauline Harris (copyeditor), and Lydia Hagen (editor). This book came to fruition through the effort of this team, and I am forever thankful for their hard work, dedication, and commitment to making it accessible to both emerging and experienced leaders.

Until next time.

Cheers!
Scott Nelson
Host of the *Higher Ground* Podcast

RECOMMENDED READING

Collins, J. (2001). Good to Great. London, England: Random House Business Books.

Deao, C. (2012). The E-Factor: How engaged patients, clinicians, leaders, and employees will transform healthcare. Gulf Breeze, FL: Fire Starter Publishing.

Greenleaf, R. K. (1997). Servant Leadership: A journey into the nature of legitimate power and greatness. Paulist Press.

University of Minnesota Editions (2016). "The Costs of Turnover" in *Human Resource Management*. Available online at: https://open.umn.edu/opentextbooks/textbooks/71

https://open.lib.umn.edu/humanresourcemanagement/chapter/7-1-the-costs-of-turnover/

Levine, D. (2021). U.S. faces crisis of burned-out health care workers. U.S. News & World Report. Retrieved from https://www.usnews.com/news/health-news/articles/2021-11-15/us-faces-crisis-of-burned-out-health-care-workers

Patterson, K., Grenny, J., McMillan, R., & Switzler, A. (2002). Crucial conversations. Maidenhead, England: McGraw-Hill Contemporary.

Studer, Q. (2003). Hardwiring Excellence: Purpose, worthwhile work, making a difference. Gulf Breeze, FL: Fire Starter Publishing.

www.ingramcontent.com/pod-product-compliance
Lightning Source LLC
La Vergne TN
LVHW022228200926
848481LV00006B/2164

* 9 7 9 8 9 9 5 3 1 3 8 0 9 *